Physical and Mental Benefits of Yoga:Nurturing Body and Mind

permitted by
copyright law.

Table of contents

Chapter 4: Yoga for Holistic Wellness

The Synergy Between Physical, Mental, and Emotional Wellness

Living a Balanced and Holistic Life

Holistic Wellness Through Yoga Practices

Chapter 5: Practical Guidance for Your Yoga Journey

Starting Your Yoga Journey: A Guide for Beginners

Tips for Practicing Yoga Safely and Effectively

Incorporating Yoga into Your Daily Routine

Setting and Achieving Your Yoga Goals

Chapter 6: The Mind-Body Connection in Yoga

The Profound Link
Between Your Body
and Mind

How Yoga Bridges the
Gap

Real-Life Applications
of the Mind-Body
Connection

Introduction

In a world that often separates the physical and the mental, the body from the mind, we invite you to embark on a holistic journey of wellness. "Physical and Mental Benefits of Yoga" is more than just an eBook; it's a guide to understanding the profound interconnectedness of our bodies and minds and how yoga serves as the bridge between them.

True wellness is an intricate tapestry woven from threads of physical health, emotional balance, and mental clarity. In this eBook, we embrace the holistic wellness approach, recognizing that our bodies and minds are not isolated entities but rather two facets of the same precious gem. We celebrate the idea that nurturing one naturally nurtures the other, creating a synergistic effect that fosters a healthier, happier, and more balanced life.

"Physical and Mental Benefits of Yoga" offers a comprehensive exploration of yoga's transformative potential. It's not just about bending your body into pretzel shapes or sitting in meditation for hours; it's about how these

practices can enhance
your physical well-
being, calm your mind,
and balance your
emotions. Here's what
you can expect from
the pages of this
eBook:

Physical Health:
Explore how yoga

enhances your strength, flexibility, and balance, and how it can be harnessed for weight management and injury prevention.

Mental Clarity: Dive into the calming waters of yoga and

learn how it reduces stress, enhances focus, and fosters mindfulness. Discover how the power of breath and meditation in yoga extends into daily life.

Emotional Balance: Uncover the

emotional stability that yoga provides, empowering you to manage anxiety, depression, and fostering self-compassion and positivity.

Holistic Wellness: Recognize that yoga

doesn't operate in silos—it's a practice that nurtures your entire being, creating a harmonious synergy between your physical, emotional, and mental health.

Practical Guidance: Gain practical tips and

insights for incorporating yoga into your daily life, whether you're a seasoned practitioner or just starting your journey.

Mind-Body Connection: Understand the

profound connection
between your body
and mind and how
yoga serves as the
bridge between these
two realms.

This eBook is your
trusted companion as
you explore the
comprehensive

benefits of yoga. It will empower you to live a healthier, happier, and more balanced life, nurturing not just your physical self but your mental and emotional well-being. Let's embark on this transformative journey together, embracing the

profound
interconnectedness of
our bodies and minds
through the ancient
practice of yoga.

Chapter 1
Yoga for Physical Health: Nurturing Your Body

In our exploration of the profound benefits of yoga, we begin with the tangible aspects of our physical health. This chapter is dedicated to understanding how yoga enhances your physical well-being, encompassing yoga poses and their physical benefits, the strengthening of your body through enhanced strength, flexibility, and balance, using yoga as a tool

for weight
management, and
how yoga can serve as
a preventive and
rehabilitative
approach for injuries.

Yoga Poses and Their Physical Benefits

Yoga is an artful science that melds movement and mindfulness. We'll delve into various yoga poses and the physical benefits they offer. From the graceful Warrior pose that enhances leg strength to the gentle Child's pose that stretches your back, each asana serves a unique purpose. You'll learn how these poses can impact your physical health and enhance your overall vitality.

Yoga is a symphony of graceful postures that

not only challenge your body but also nurture it. In this chapter, we'll embark on a journey through various yoga poses and explore the unique physical benefits each one offers. These poses are not merely exercises but gateways to enhancing your physical well-being.

Warrior Pose (Virabhadrasana)

Physical Benefits:

Strengthens the legs: The Warrior Pose series, especially Warrior I and II, are renowned for enhancing leg strength. These poses engage the quadriceps, hamstrings, and calf muscles, promoting muscular endurance.

Improves balance: By holding these stances and focusing on your alignment, you enhance your balance and concentration.

Stretches the hips: The wide stance of Warrior poses opens up the hips and groin area, promoting flexibility and reducing stiffness.

Downward Dog Pose (Adho Mukha Svanasana)

Physical Benefits:

Strengthens the arms and shoulders: Downward Dog is a powerful pose that builds upper body strength. It engages the deltoids, triceps, and the muscles of the upper back.

Stretches the hamstrings and calves: It provides an intense

stretch for the posterior chain of your legs, promoting flexibility and reducing tightness.

Aligns the spine: This pose encourages proper spinal alignment, helping to alleviate back pain and improving posture.

Cobra Pose (Bhujangasana)

Physical Benefits:

Strengthens the back: Cobra pose targets the muscles of the

lower back, helping to build strength and resilience.

Enhances flexibility: This pose opens the chest and stretches the abdominal muscles, promoting flexibility in the front of the body.

Relieves tension: Cobra pose can alleviate tension in the lower back and help improve overall spinal health.

Tree Pose (Vrikshasana)

Physical Benefits:

Enhances balance: Tree pose challenges your balance, requiring you to engage your core and stabilize your body.

Strengthens the legs and ankles: Balancing on one leg strengthens the leg muscles and the muscles around the ankles.

Improves posture: Practicing Tree pose encourages you to stand tall and align your spine properly, thus improving posture.

Child's Pose (Balasana)

Physical Benefits:

Relaxes the back and shoulders: Child's pose is a restorative posture that relaxes the back and shoulders, reducing tension.

Stretches the hips and thighs: By sitting back on your heels and extending your arms forward, you stretch the hips and thighs.

Relieves lower back pain: This pose can be soothing for lower back discomfort and is often used as a resting position during yoga practice.

Each of these yoga poses offers a unique set of physical benefits. By incorporating a variety of poses into your practice, you can strengthen, stretch, and support your body in various ways. Remember that the physical benefits of yoga extend beyond the mat, promoting overall physical health and well-being.

Enhancing Strength, Flexibility, and Balance

Yoga is a harmonious blend of physical strength, flexibility, and balance. Through a range of poses and sequences, it nurtures these attributes, creating a harmonious equilibrium within your body. We'll explore how yoga empowers you to build physical strength, enhance flexibility in muscles and joints, and improve balance, which is essential for both physical and mental well-being.

Using Yoga for Weight Management

Yoga is not merely about the postures you strike on a mat; it extends into the management of your body weight. Discover how yoga can be harnessed as a tool for weight management. We'll explore yoga's impact on metabolism, appetite regulation, and how it fosters mindful eating. This chapter provides insights into how yoga can be an ally in your journey to a healthy weight.

Preventing and Managing Injuries with Yoga

Injuries are a part of life, but yoga can be a powerful means of both prevention and rehabilitation. We'll delve into the preventive aspects of yoga, including how it can improve your posture, alignment, and overall body awareness. Additionally, we'll discuss how yoga serves as a healing modality for injuries, providing gentle techniques and practices that facilitate recovery.

Chapter 2
Yoga for Mental Clarity: The Path to Inner Peace

As we delve into the world of yoga, we transition from the realm of the physical to the boundless landscape of the mind.

This chapter is dedicated to the myriad ways in which yoga fosters mental clarity, offering insight into the vast mental benefits it provides. From calming the mind and reducing stress to enhancing focus, mindfulness, and the profound power of breath and meditation, this chapter is your guide to embracing a calm and focused mental state through yoga.

The Mental Benefits of Yoga

Yoga is not just a practice of the body but also a sanctuary for the mind. We'll explore the diverse mental benefits that yoga provides, including:

Stress Reduction: The practice of yoga

creates a tranquil
space in which you
can leave behind the
chaos of daily life and
embrace a calm,
stress-free state.

Emotional Balance:
Yoga empowers you
to manage your
emotions effectively,

enhancing emotional resilience and promoting a sense of inner peace.

Mental Clarity: The stillness of the yoga practice allows you to find clarity and insight, often leading to creative and problem-solving breakthroughs.

Improved Concentration: Yoga refines your concentration skills, allowing you to focus with greater precision and depth.

Calming the Mind and Reducing Stress

In the hustle and bustle of life, the mind often becomes a turbulent sea of thoughts. Yoga offers a life raft, guiding you to calm the mind and reduce stress. We'll explore how various yoga practices, including gentle asanas and restorative poses, help to soothe the nervous system and reduce stress.

Enhancing Focus and Mindfulness

In an age of constant distractions, the ability to focus and be present is a precious gift. Yoga nurtures your focus and mindfulness, allowing you to fully engage with the present moment. We'll delve into mindfulness

practices and discuss
how yoga enhances
your ability to remain
attentive and engaged
in everyday life.

The Power of Breath
and Meditation

Yoga places tremendous importance on the breath and meditation. We'll discuss the profound effects of controlled breathing techniques and the transformative power of meditation. These practices, deeply rooted in yoga, are tools for finding inner peace, reducing anxiety, and promoting mental clarity.

This chapter invites you to explore the mental landscape of yoga, discovering how it calms the mind, reduces stress, enhances focus and mindfulness, and empowers you through the profound practices of breath and meditation. The benefits of yoga extend far beyond the physical realm, creating a deep sense of mental clarity and serenity. As we continue our journey, you'll find practical insights and techniques to apply these mental benefits to your daily life, fostering a sense of calm and focus that permeates your existence.

Chapter 3

Yoga for Emotional Balance: Nurturing Your Heart and Soul

In our ongoing exploration of yoga, we now venture into the realm of emotions and the profound role that yoga plays in fostering emotional balance. This chapter is dedicated to understanding the ways in which yoga promotes emotional stability, its role in managing conditions like anxiety and depression, and how it fosters self-compassion, positivity,

and emotional release
and healing.

Emotional Stability Through Yoga

Emotional turbulence is an intrinsic part of life, and yoga provides a safe harbor to navigate these waters.

We'll explore the profound ways in which yoga nurtures emotional stability, including:

Mind-Body Connection: Understanding how the connection between your body

and mind impacts
your emotional state.

Emotional Awareness:
Recognizing and
acknowledging your
emotions as they arise.

Release of Tension:
Yoga practices that
allow you to release

emotional tension stored in the body.

Managing Anxiety and Depression

Anxiety and depression are challenges faced by many, and yoga offers valuable tools for managing these conditions. We'll delve into how yoga can be used as a complementary approach to conventional treatments, including:

Breathing Techniques: The use of specific

breathwork to reduce anxiety and enhance relaxation.

Mindfulness Practices: Techniques to foster present-moment awareness and alleviate symptoms of depression and anxiety.

Empowerment: How yoga empowers individuals to regain control over their emotional well-being.

Fostering Self-Compassion and Positivity

Yoga is not just about physical postures; it's a journey of self-discovery and self-compassion. We'll explore how yoga empowers individuals to be kinder to themselves, fostering self-compassion, self-love, and positivity.

You'll discover how positive affirmations, mindfulness, and the yoga philosophy contribute to this transformation.

Emotional Release and Healing

Yoga provides a sacred space for emotional release and healing. We'll delve into practices that allow individuals to release pent-up emotions and embark on a journey of healing, including:

Yoga for Emotional Release: Specific poses and sequences that facilitate emotional release.

Emotional Healing: How the yoga practice nurtures emotional healing and recovery.

Art of Letting Go:
Techniques for letting go of past emotional burdens and embracing a brighter, more emotionally balanced future.

This chapter invites you to explore the emotional facets of

yoga, understanding how it nurtures emotional stability, empowers individuals to manage conditions like anxiety and depression, fosters self-compassion and positivity, and provides a path to emotional release and healing. The benefits

of yoga extend
beyond the physical
and mental, creating a
deep sense of
emotional balance
and well-being. As we
continue our journey,
you'll find practical
insights and
techniques to apply
these emotional
benefits to your daily

life, fostering
emotional harmony
and resilience.

Chapter 4

Yoga for Holistic Wellness: The Path to Wholeness

Yoga, as we've discovered, is not just a practice of physical postures or mental clarity. It is a holistic journey that intertwines the realms of the physical, mental, and emotional, nurturing a sense of wholeness and balance. In this chapter, we explore the profound synergy between physical, mental, and emotional wellness, delve into the art of living a balanced and holistic life, and uncover how yoga practices serve as the conduit to holistic well-being.

The Synergy Between Physical, Mental, and Emotional Wellness

Wellness is not a one-dimensional concept but a multidimensional tapestry that weaves physical, mental, and emotional threads together. We'll explore the profound synergy between these dimensions, understanding how they interconnect and influence one another. Recognize that your physical health impacts your mental and emotional well-being and vice versa. Discover how yoga acts as a bridge between these facets of wellness, creating a harmonious whole.

Living a Balanced and Holistic Life

Living a balanced life is an art, and yoga provides the canvas for this masterpiece. We'll delve into the principles of balanced living, which include:

Mindful Choices:
Making conscious
decisions that align
with your physical,
mental, and
emotional well-being.

Prioritizing Self-Care:
Recognizing the
importance of self-

care to nourish your entire being.

Wellness as a Lifestyle: Embracing wellness as a lifelong journey rather than a temporary goal.

Holistic Wellness Through Yoga Practices

Yoga is not a standalone practice but an approach to living that nurtures holistic wellness. We'll explore how various yoga practices,

including asanas
(physical postures),
pranayama (breath
control), and
meditation, can be
harnessed to nurture
holistic well-being.
These practices
empower individuals
to integrate physical,
mental, and

emotional wellness into their daily lives.

This chapter invites you to embark on a journey toward holistic wellness through yoga. We'll explore the profound synergy between physical, mental, and emotional well-being, recognizing that the tapestry of wellness is multi-dimensional. By learning to live a balanced and holistic life and applying yoga practices that encompass your entire being, you empower yourself to experience the full spectrum of well-being. As we continue our journey, you'll find practical insights and techniques to apply these holistic wellness principles to your daily life, fostering a sense of wholeness and balance that

enriches your
existence.

Chapter 5

Practical Guidance for Your Yoga Journey: Navigating the Path with Confidence

As you embark on your yoga journey, this chapter offers practical guidance to ensure you navigate the path with confidence. Whether you're a seasoned practitioner or a beginner, it's essential to have a roadmap that leads to a fulfilling and effective yoga practice. We'll provide insights on how to start your yoga journey, tips for practicing yoga safely and effectively, incorporating yoga into your daily routine, and setting and achieving your yoga goals.

Starting Your Yoga Journey: A Guide for Beginners

For those who are new to yoga, this section is your gateway to a successful start. You'll discover:

Selecting the Right Class: How to choose the style of yoga that best aligns with your goals and needs.

Essential Equipment: An overview of the basic yoga equipment you'll need.

Creating a Home Practice: Tips for practicing at home,

especially when attending a class isn't feasible.

Tips for Practicing Yoga Safely and Effectively

Safety and effectiveness are paramount in your

yoga practice. We'll delve into:

Warm-Up and Cool-Down: The importance of proper preparation and recovery in your practice.

Yoga Etiquette:
Guidelines for
practicing respect and
mindfulness in a
group class.

**Listening to Your
Body:** How to
recognize your body's
signals and practice
safely.

Incorporating Yoga into Your Daily Routine

Yoga isn't merely a practice but a way of life. We'll explore how to integrate yoga into your daily routine, including:

Morning and Evening Rituals: How to create simple, yet meaningful, yoga practices for the start and end of your day.

Desk Yoga: Techniques to alleviate the strain of

sedentary work with desk-friendly yoga.

Family and Group Yoga: Ways to involve loved ones in your practice, fostering a sense of community and shared well-being.

Setting and Achieving Your Yoga Goals

Goals provide direction and motivation on your yoga journey. We'll guide you through:

Identifying Your Goals: Defining what you

wish to achieve
through your practice,
whether it's increased
flexibility, stress
reduction, or spiritual
growth.

**Goal Setting
Techniques:**
Strategies for setting

clear, achievable, and meaningful goals.

Tracking Progress: How to monitor your development and celebrate your successes.

This chapter is your compass, helping you

navigate your yoga journey effectively, safely, and with purpose. Whether you're new to yoga or a seasoned practitioner, the practical guidance provided here ensures that your practice aligns with your goals and becomes an integral part of your daily life. As we continue our journey, you'll find the tools and support needed to unlock the transformative potential of yoga and nurture holistic wellness.

Chapter 6

The Mind-Body Connection in Yoga: Bridging the Gap for Holistic Wellness

In the world of yoga, the relationship between the body and mind is profound and intrinsic. This chapter delves into the profound link between your body and mind, how yoga serves as the bridge that connects these two facets of your being, and real-life applications of the mind-body connection. Understanding this connection is essential for achieving holistic wellness through yoga.

The Profound Link Between Your Body and Mind

The body and mind are not separate entities but intricately

intertwined. We'll explore:

Emotions and Physical Sensations: How emotions can manifest as physical sensations and vice versa.

Stress and Tension: The connection

between mental stress and physical tension in the body.

The Power of Awareness: The role of awareness in recognizing the mind-body connection.

How Yoga Bridges the Gap

Yoga is a masterful bridge between the body and mind, offering a space for their harmonious interaction. We'll uncover:

Breath as a Link: How conscious breath control and regulation serve as a vital link between your body and mind.

Yoga Poses: The physical postures that encourage the mind-body connection

through alignment
and awareness.

Meditation and Mindfulness: The profound practices of meditation and mindfulness that anchor the mind in the present moment.

Real-Life Applications of the Mind-Body Connection

The mind-body connection isn't confined to the mat but extends into all aspects of life. We'll explore:

Stress Management: How yoga techniques can be applied to reduce stress and its physical manifestations.

Emotional Regulation: Strategies for using the mind-body connection to manage

and transform
emotions.

Enhanced Well-Being:
Real-life examples of
individuals who have
harnessed the mind-
body connection for
greater well-being.

This chapter invites you to explore the mind-body connection that's intrinsic to yoga, understanding how it bridges the gap between your physical and mental well-being. As you deepen your understanding of this connection, you'll find that yoga serves as the conduit for nurturing a harmonious synergy between your body and mind. This harmony extends beyond the mat, enriching your entire life with holistic wellness. As we continue our journey, you'll find practical insights and techniques to apply the mind-body connection to your daily life, fostering a sense of unity and balance.